TRISTAN TEAPOT SERIES

BOOK FOUR

Jasmine Tea

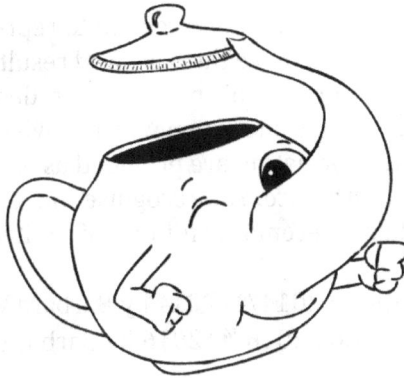

Barbi Wildish

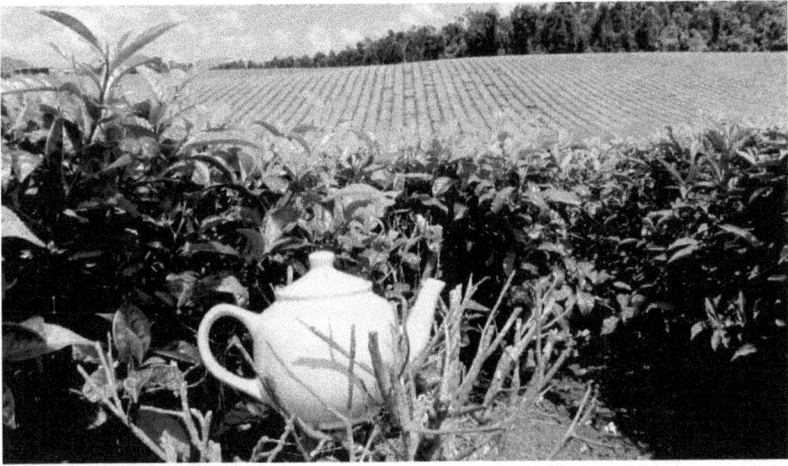

Jasmine Tea

Tristan Teapot resting and admiring
Nucifora Tea Plantation
Atherton Tablelands, Australia

If you have health, you have wealth

Table of Contents

What is
- Oolong Jasmine Tea
- White Jasmine Tea
- Black Jasmine Tea
- Vanilla, Rose and Orange – Another Dimension

How Do They Grade Tea
- Jasmine Tea
- Black Tea
- Green Tea
- Oolong Tea
- White Tea

What Makes For A Quality Tea Experience
- What is the best way to have a quality tea experience
- What are the benefits of high quality tea
- How is quality ensured
- There are a number of factors in a high quality tea Offering
- Tea Cupping

What Is Jasmine Tea?

One of the tea blends you simply cannot miss is Jasmine tea.

If you have never tried it, you're missing a real treat. Much of the world has already discovered the fragrance and flavour of Jasmine tea. In fact, it is the most popular Chinese flavoured tea.

Jasmine tea is made from a special blend of high quality loose tea leaves with jasmine petals added. The jasmine petals impart a delicate yet very aromatic fragrance to the tea, and also impart a slightly sweet flavour.

Jasmine has been produced in China for at least 700 years. The original production of the tea included plucking the jasmine blossoms, and when the blossoms began to release their fragrance, they add them to the tea leaves at night, to ensure the best infusion of the aroma and fragrance.

In most cases, the tea was scented twice using two different sets of jasmine blossoms to ensure that the tea was properly infused.

Jasmine green tea is one of the healthiest teas you can drink.

Today, most jasmine tea is still made with green tea, though the process is no longer carried out by hand. Most believe that the Fujian region of China produces the best jasmine tea because it is this area of China, that produces the largest and most heavily scented jasmine blossoms and the loosest green tea leaves.

Green tea has been shown to have more health benefits than black tea because of the way it is processed. Green tea does not go through a fermentation process. The fermentation process that happens to black tea converts the natural anti-oxidants to other compounds. So, while black tea is a healthy beverage, it is not as healthy as green tea, whose anti-oxidants are left in their natural state.

Anti-oxidants are important to protecting our health. Anti-oxidants help to neutralize free radicals. Free radicals are oxygen containing molecules that are created as a by product of converting the food we eat into energy. Left

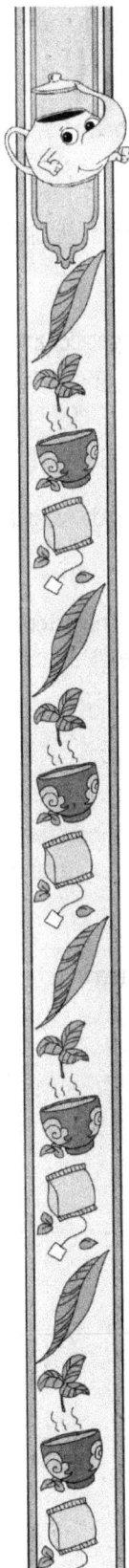

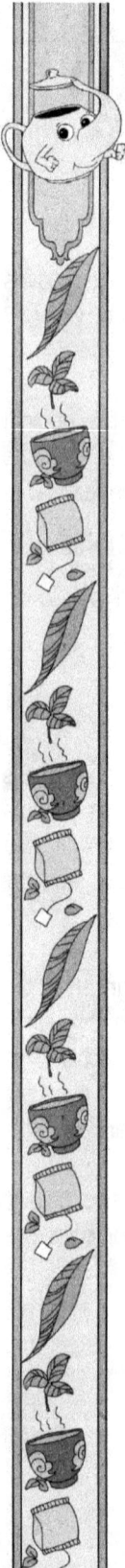

unchecked, these free radicals damage our cells and DNA, leading to aging and dis-ease.

A diet rich in anti-oxidants keeps these free radicals under control. And, green tea is one of the best sources of anti-oxidants around.

Including green tea in your diet along with other plant based products like fruits and vegetables can help protect your health.

In recent years, a lot of research has shown some very specific and interesting things about drinking green tea. We've learned that green tea has the power to prevent many types of cancer, including breast, colon and lung cancer.

In addition, long term green tea drinkers tend to have a lower body weight and are more successful at losing weight.

Green tea can also help prevent heart dis-ease by helping lower cholesterol and preventing blood clots, which are the leading cause of heart attacks and strokes.

In addition, green tea is helpful at regulating insulin naturally.

So, if you like the idea of adding green tea to your diet, then jasmine green tea may be a great way to enjoy a wonderful fragrance and flavour and protect your health at the same time.

If, however, you're not a green tea drinker, you can find jasmine tea in other forms.

JASMINE TEA DATES BACK TO THE SUNG DYNASTY

The looser the tea leaves, the better they are able to absorb the jasmine fragrance. The first plucking of green tea will produce the best jasmine tea because the leaves are at their tenderest.

While the majority of jasmine tea is green tea, there are also quite a few white and oolong jasmine teas. White tea, in particular, lends itself quite well to being combined with jasmine because both offer a sweet and subtle flavour and fragrance.

Oolong jasmine teas are smooth with the fruity taste that is common in oolong tea. However, the jasmine also makes the tea fragrant and sweet. You'll find oolong jasmine tea to have one of the most distinctive flavours of any jasmine tea.

And, for the die hard black tea drinker, there is also black jasmine tea which can be a bit harder to find than other varieties of jasmine tea. Because black tea has a stronger flavour, the jasmine flavour is less noticeable when it is combined with black tea. Still many black tea lovers who favour lightly flavoured teas find this blend very appealing.

• Brewing the perfect cuppa

Regardless of the variety of jasmine tea you choose, you should make the time and effort to brew the tea correctly to ensure the best flavour.

First, Begin with the best loose tea. The best way to ensure that you get good tea is to purchase it from a reputable tea shop, whether in your local area or online. Really good tea may cost a bit more, but its quality is unmistakable.

Second, Brewing good tea requires fresh cold water. Put the water in a clean tea kettle and bring it to a boil on the stove.

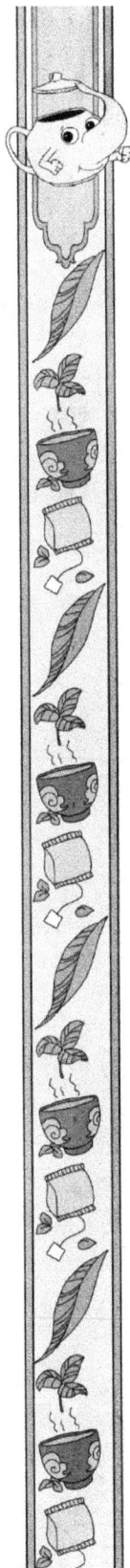

9

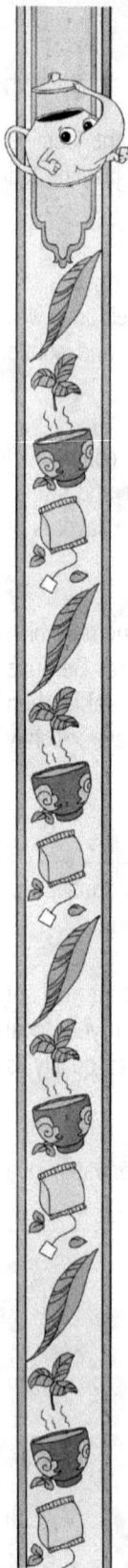

Third, Meanwhile, put hot tap water in your teapot to warm it up while the water is heating. Once the water boils, remove the tap water from your pot and add your tea leaves.

Quantity, For white jasmine tea, use about 2 teaspoons of loose tea per cup.
For other jasmine teas, you'll only need about 1 teaspoon per cup.

Follow the table below to choose the appropriate water temperature and steeping time for your jasmine tea:

• Water Temperature/Steeping time for the varieties:

Adhering to the appropriate water temperature and steeping time is critical for making good tea.

Too much steeping and your tea will be bitter; too little and the tea will be thin and weak. Water that is too hot for delicate teas like green and white will compromise the teas light flavour.

• Iced Tea

Jasmine tea, particularly green and white jasmine teas, are also wonderful as iced tea. The jasmine fragrance and light sweetness are perfect for a hot day.

To make iced tea, brew several servings of tea at once and cool. For white and green teas, allow the tea to cool completely before you add ice. Adding ice to the hot tea may dilute the delicate flavour too much, making it taste weak and flavourless.

• Soothing and a Delicious Beverage

Jasmine tea has been around for centuries for a reason. It's one of the most delicious varieties of flavoured tea around, regardless of the type of tea used. Whether you choose black, white, oolong or green jasmine tea, you're sure to be delighted by its fragrant bouquet and its sweet taste. It

Black Jasmine	Boiling	3-5 minutes	complim
White Jasmine	185 deg F	5-8 minutes	ents
Green Jasmine	160 deg F	1-2 minutes	every
Oolong Jasmine	Boiling	2-3 minutes	flavour

of tea and creates a soothing and delicious beverage whether hot or cold. And jasmine tea is a healthy beverage, too.

In recent years, tea, particularly green and white teas have received a lot of attention for their potent anti-oxidants. The anti-oxidants in tea and other plant based foods help fight free radicals in our bodies.

These free radicals are oxygen containing molecules that damage our cells and DNA. A diet rich in anti-oxidants rid our bodies of these free radicals before they can damage our bodies. Diets rich in green and white tea have been shown to prevent serious illness like cancer, high cholesterol and diabetes.

It is good for you so try some, I'm sure you'll be pleased.

HOW IS JASMINE TEA DIFFERENT FROM OTHER TEAS

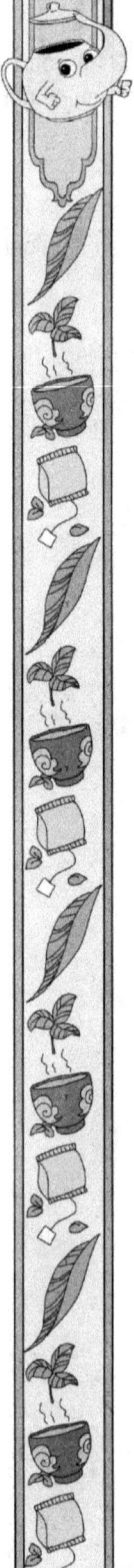

If you're a tea drinker, it's likely you have tried jasmine tea. Jasmine tea is the most popular blend of Chinese tea, and has been produced for more than 700 years.

It was first produced during the Sung dynasty, by plucking the jasmine leaves as soon as they begin to bloom.

The freshly plucked jasmine leaves were stored in a cool place until nightfall, when the blossoms began to release their fragrance. Then the jasmine petals were added to dry heaps of tea leaves, to allow the dry tea leaves to absorb the fragrance. Ordinary grades were scented two or three times; the special grades even more. Today, the process is much the same, though it may not be carried out by hand these days.

The best jasmine tea is said to come from the Fujian province in China. This is because this area of China produces the largest and heaviest scented jasmine leaves and some of the loosest tea leaves, which can absorb the jasmine fragrance better.

Like with most other teas, the first plucking in the spring produce the very best jasmine tea because the tea leaves are so tender. It is sometimes referred to as Spring Breeze jasmine tea.

Jasmine tea has been the favourite tea of those in northern China for many years, but has gained favour all over the world in more recent years. There are some interesting facts and differences about jasmine tea.

It was believed to have spiritual powers. That is why jasmine tea became so popular for tea ceremonies.

Jasmine tea is made from green, oolong, white or black tea. You can find it in your favourite variety of tea.

12

• Which Jasmine tea should I choose?

So, if you're in the market for jasmine tea, which should you choose?

Experiment by combining jasmine tea with other teas. You may find the other teas that don't really appeal to you in their plainest form but are very appealing when combined with jasmine.
Here are some characteristics of the different varieties of jasmine tea.

• Jasmine Green Tea

This is the most common form of Jasmine tea. Jasmine green tea has a very natural and light flavour, with the plant taste of green tea complemented by the sweet and fragrant jasmine blossoms.

What makes jasmine green tea so healthy is that it retains the tea's anti-oxidants in their most natural form, because the tea is not fermented.

These natural anti-oxidants protect our health by neutralizing the free radicals in our bodies. These free radicals, which are created during our digestive process, can damage our cells and DNA if we don't keep them in check. A diet rich in anti-oxidants like those found in green and white tea keeps these free radicals under control.

• Oolong Jasmine Tea

Is likely the second most common form of green tea. Oolong teas are semi-fermented, meaning that they are fermented for a shorter period of time than black teas. To produce a oolong tea, fermentation must be stopped when the leaves are 30% red and 70% green.

It is the ability to stop the fermentation at precisely the right time that gives oolong teas their distinct flavour. Most oolong teas are dried using charcoal, giving it another distinct dimension. Oolong jasmine teas are smooth with the fruity taste that is common in oolong tea. However, the jasmine also makes the tea fragrant and sweet.

13

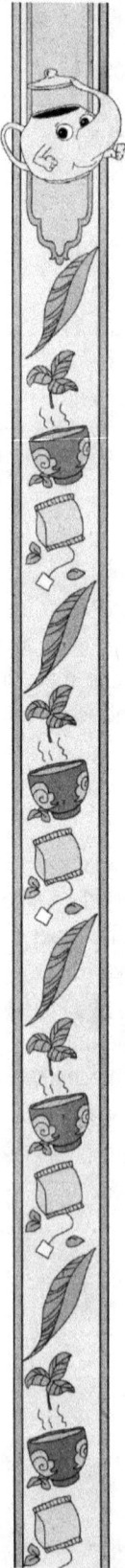

• White Jasmine Tea

The combination of light and sweet white tea with fragrant jasmine makes for a very delicate flavour. As white tea gains popularity in the Western world, it's likely that white jasmine tea will become easier to find. Because white tea, like green tea, is unfermented, you will gain the same health benefits from drinking white tea that green tea provides.

• Black Jasmine Tea

While black tea is the most common variety of tea consumed in the Western world, it is the tea least commonly combined with jasmine. Black tea is bolder and stronger than green and white teas, so the jasmine is not as prominent in the flavour or aroma.

Regardless of the variety of tea you choose, it's likely you'll find that the addition of jasmine is a true delight.

Most tea drinkers find the scent of jasmine tea very soothing, making it a great tea to enjoy in the evening.

You're certain to want to sample many varieties of jasmine tea to determine your favourites.

If you love the fragrance and sweetness of jasmine combined with tea as much as I do, you'll have a favourite jasmine tea from every tea variety available!

I love going for Yum-cha and as soon as I sit down, I order a pot of Jasmine Tea. I find it aids in the digestion of my meal. I love it.

- ## Oolong Jasmine Tea

Oolong jasmine tea is also a very popular blend. Oolong teas are also processed a bit differently than black teas.

It is semi-fermented, meaning that they are fermented, but for a shorter period of time than black teas. To produce a good oolong tea, fermentation must be stopped when the leaves are 30% red and 70% green.

It is the ability to stop the fermentation at precisely the right time that gives oolong tea its distinct flavour. Most are also dried using charcoal, giving it another distinct dimension. It has the typically smooth and fruity taste usually found in oolong teas combined with the fragrant sweetness of jasmine.

- ## White Jasmine Tea

Jasmine tea can be made from white tea, too.

In fact, today, white jasmine tea is becoming quite popular.

It is a sweet and light white tea combined with the subtle scent of jasmine making for a very delicate and refreshing beverage.

It is one of the mildest jasmine teas you'll find. And, drinking white jasmine tea will provide all the health benefits of drinking green jasmine tea.

- ## Black Jasmine Tea

Finally, there are also a few black jasmine teas. Because black tea has a bolder flavour, you'll find black jasmine teas to have a more subtle jasmine flavour, as the jasmine scent and taste does not stand out as much when combined with black tea as it does when combined with lighter green and oolong teas.

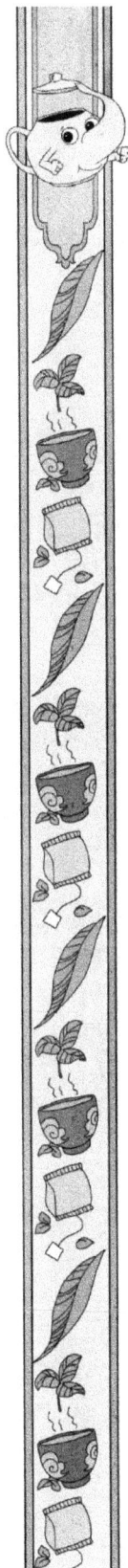

15

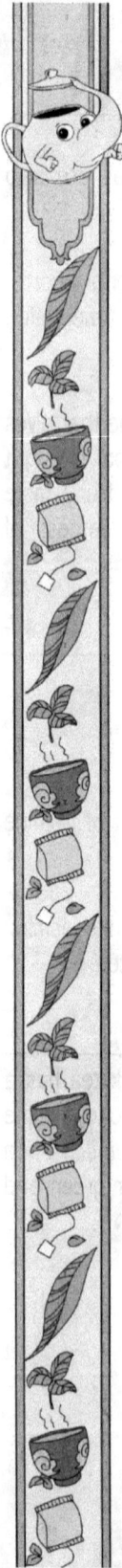

As you can see, jasmine is a favourite for blending with tea, making jasmine tea one of the easiest tea blends to find.

Because jasmine tea is so common, it is important to ensure that you're choosing only the best quality tea when you purchase it.

The best jasmine tea is made using real jasmine petals combined with the highest quality loose leaf teas. You'll often find that some of the best and most flavourful jasmine teas use tightly rolled green tea pearls mixed with jasmine petals.

In addition to teas mixed only with jasmine, you'll also find jasmine tea mixed with other flavours as well.

Because it imparts mostly fragrance and only a subtle flavour to the tea, it mixes easily with other flavours, as well.

• Vanilla, Rose and Orange – Another Dimension

You'll find jasmine tea flavoured also with vanilla, rose and orange. All of these have the delicate aroma and sweet flavour of jasmine, but include a second, complementary flavour to add dimension to the taste of your tea experience. Whatever form of jasmine tea you choose, you're sure to love it.

Jasmine tea, whether in green, oolong or black form is one of the most traditional of all Chinese teas and certainly one of the most fragrant and enjoyable.

16

- ## Jasmine Tea

Jasmine tea is the most popular flavoured tea in the world. The first jasmine tea was produced in China and made from green tea. Today, however, jasmine flowers are used to scent teas from all over the world, in black, white, green and oolong varieties.

What makes jasmine tea so wonderful is its special blend of high quality loose tea leaves with jasmine petals. The jasmine petals impart a delicate yet very aromatic fragrance and a slightly sweet flavour to the tea.

Jasmine has been produced in China for at least 700 years. The original production of jasmine tea included plucking the jasmine blossoms just as they were beginning to open in the morning. Then the jasmine petals were kept cool until evening when they were added to the green tea leaves.

The jasmine petals were infused with the tea leaves at night because this is the time when the petals release their fragrance. The teas were infused with the jasmine petals multiple times to obtain just the right scent and flavour. Today, the process is more automated, but good quality jasmine tea still depends upon using the best loose tea and infusing it with just the right amount of jasmine blossom.

For the jasmine lover, there are many choices in tea. However, it can be difficult to spot a really good jasmine tea, because interpreting the way teas are graded can be difficult.

First, it's important to understand that there are no international standards on grading tea. Each country uses their own system, and even different types of tea are graded differently. For example, green teas are not graded the same as white teas.

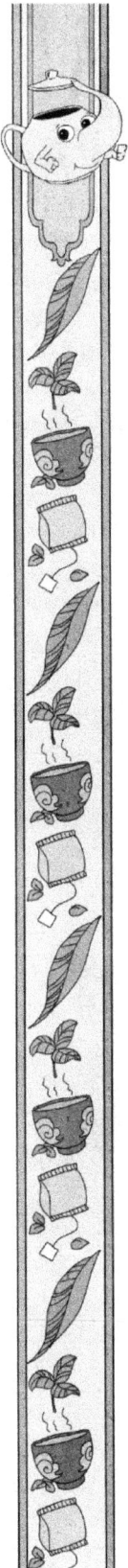

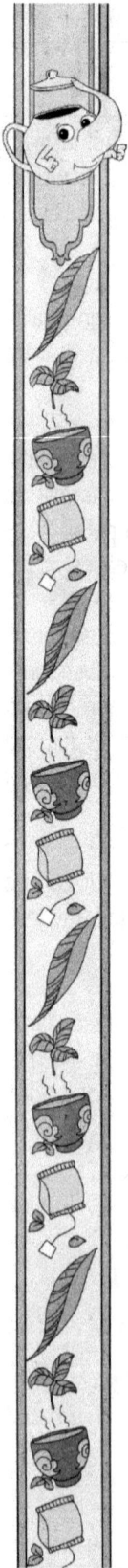

So, understanding how the jasmine tea you are considering is graded, really means understanding how the tea variety that the jasmine tea is made from is graded. Here are some examples to help make it easier to understand.

- **Black Tea**

Black tea is graded primarily based on how it is processed. So, while this will tell you the approximate percentage of whole leaves in your tea, and may tell you if it comes from an early or late plucking, it's not the total picture when it comes to judging the quality of the tea.

Knowing where the tea was grown and how tea is harvested in this part of the world is important, too. In the US, the best black teas are considered whole leaf teas and are designated by the term Tippy Golden Flowery Orange Pekoe.

You should avoid teas marked 'dust', as these are typically the lowest grades of black tea.

- **Green Tea**

Green tea is typically graded by the shape of the leaf in China. In other parts of the world, green tea is also usually graded by leaf shape, but different names are used to describe the leaf shapes.

Within the leaf shapes, in both China and other countries, you will find grades that further break down the quality of the tea.

- **Oolong Tea**

Oolong tea from China is graded in a simple manner that is easy to follow and understand. The best oolong tea is referred to as 'Fanciest' or 'Extra Fancy', while the lowest grade of oolong tea is referred to as 'Common'.

Since most oolong tea is produced in China, it is fairly simple to sort out a good oolong jasmine tea. However, if you buy an oolong tea from another country it could be graded in a totally different manner.

• White Tea

White tea's grading is somewhat simpler, because when the tea leaves are plucked, it is not part of determining the quality. All white tea is from a first plucking, because there is only one plucking of white tea during each growing season.

Therefore, choosing a quality white jasmine tea from China simply means choosing one of the two highest grades of white tea, Silver Needles or White Peony.

However, if you choose a white Ceylon jasmine tea or a white Darjeeling jasmine tea, the grading will be totally different.

To choose a good jasmine tea, begin by determining whether you want a white, green, black or oolong jasmine tea.
If you are new to drinking jasmine tea, it's likely best to begin with a Chinese green jasmine tea, as this tea represents the true essence of the jasmine tea.

Once you've sorted out the variety of tea you'd like to try and the country of the tea's origin, simply look for this tea from a quality tea store.

If you can't find the combination you have chosen at a good tea store, then it's likely that very good quality of this particular combination will be difficult to find.

Keep looking until you find a combination that can be purchased from a reputable tea supplier. This way you will be assured of the quality of the tea, even if the combination was not what you had originally planned.

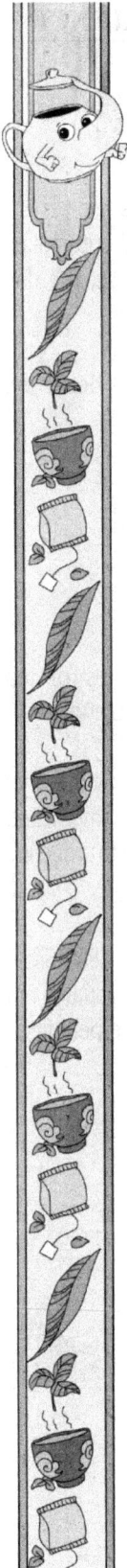

WHAT MAKES FOR A QUALITY TEA EXPERIENCE

Tea is more than a beverage. It is a way of life that leads to well-being and satisfaction, and it is healthy and tastes good as well.

To start the day with a steaming cup of your favourite tea puts the rest of the day in a better perspective, and to end that day with a final cup makes the experience so much better. In the mind of many tea drinkers, the day just seems better with tea in it.

It only follows therefore, that the higher the quality of the tea, the better the experience.

- **What is the best way to have a quality tea experience?**

First, start with tea that you like.

Although tea comes from one plant, there are many varieties of tea depending on how it is processed and whether it is flavoured or blended.

Country of origin is also important. In addition tea is grown in many areas of the world under varying conditions so environmental forces are important. Chose a quality tea that not only tastes good, but leaves one with a feeling of wellness and contentment.

From quality comes satisfaction and there are many levels of quality. Since tea is a commodity, the price you pay for high quality is usually not significantly more than low quality tea, particularly considering the benefits.

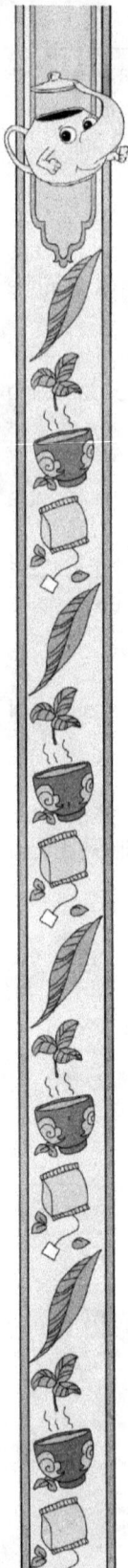

• What are the benefits of high quality tea?

First the flavour should be satisfying and memorable with a light but unique taste that is pleasant and satisfying.

Next the tea should enhance good health in the drinker. Fresh, quality tea can reduce stress and minimize the effects of free radicals, thus promoting an aura of good health.

Quality tea also promotes a tea lifestyle where the drinker makes tea an important and healthy part of their life and that life becomes stress free and enjoyable.

Tea is also a very adaptable drink that can be served hot or cold depending on the ambient temperature and it can also serve as a cooking medium.

There are many recipes for cooking with tea. My Recipe Book:

No Tea In My Cheesecake, Thank You

has tea in every recipe! Delicious – check it out today.

Remember that the benefits are enhanced as the quality increases and loose, whole leaf tea is often preferred by knowledgeable tea drinkers.

• How is Quality Ensured?

There are two important elements in ensuring a quality tea experience:

1. Quality of the tea and
2. Quality of the preparation.

Quality of the tea is part and parcel of purchasing tea from a supplier with a culture of quality.

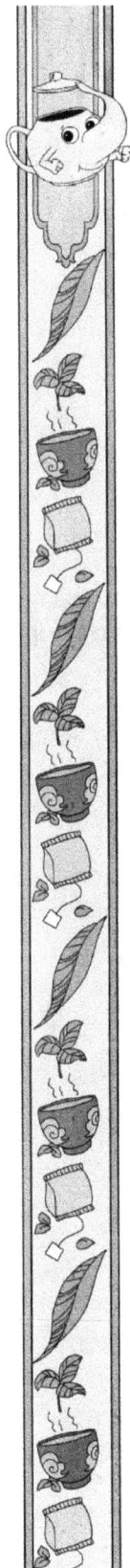

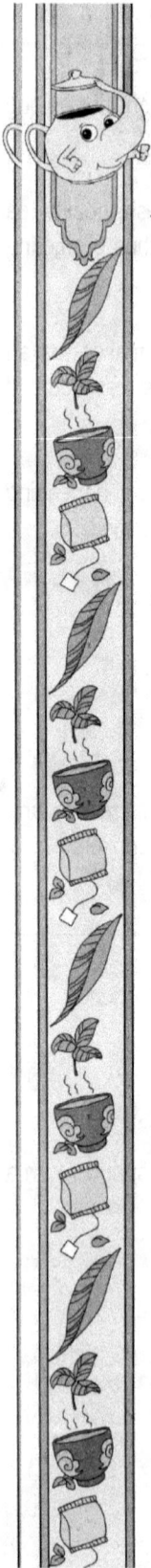

Since individual shipment of tea from the exporting tea garden can and do vary in quality, deal with an importer who tastes each shipment as part of an overall quality control program.

- **There are a number of factors in a high quality tea offering:**

ï   Location and reputation of the tea garden

ï   Environmental factors such at temperature and humidity

ï   Time of the year for tea plucking

ï   Quality of processing

ï   Blending/ recipe for flavoured and blended tea

Tea cupping of each shipment by the supplier will ensure consistent high quality.

Quality of preparation is as much of an art as it is a science, but the elements of preparation is to use bottled water of high quality (purified water is best) and steep the brew not more than four minutes in order to avoid bitterness from the release of tannic acid.
Serve in high quality tea ware with good friends, and the experience will be memorable.

- **Tea Cupping**

Cupping is the most important of all tea trade procedures after growing and
It is essential to buying tea and assessing its usefulness at every level of

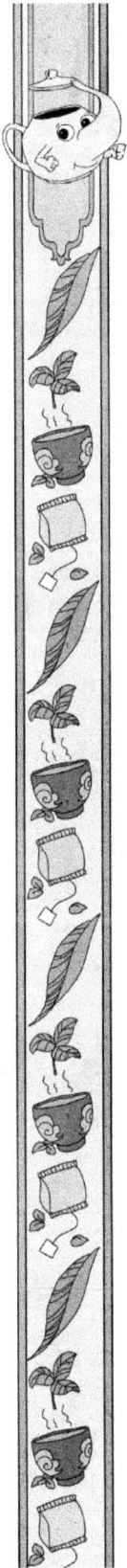

the trade; tea professionals often cup dozens of teas in a line at a single go.

Cupping is not just tasting, but examination for purposes of comparison and contrast. Consistency is the key. You have to follow the same procedure every time you cup, using identical lighting, equipment, water, temperature of water, weight of dry leaf, length of steeping time, and ritual practices right down to always cupping at the same time of day and in a calm state of mind.

All you need is a clean, well-lighted area perfectly free from odours, a set of **tasting cups** with lids, a kettle, a gram scale, a timer, **tea trays** and spoons.

Packages of tea are lined up , along with tea trays holding dry leaf from each sample; in front of these, lined up are tasting cups.

Now they measure out an exact two grams of each sample and put it into the cup. They then go down the line and fill each cup with steaming to boiling water and set the timer for the appropriate time based on tea.

When time is up, they follow the same order in tipping the cups so as to drain the tea liquor into the tasting bowl. They then go down the line again and empty the infused tea leaf onto cup lids and place them atop the cups.

Finally, they proceed down the line with their spoon, slurping a spoonful of each tea with a sudden (and inevitably loud) in-take so that the tea sprays the entire interior of the mouth.

inspect a specimen of both its dry leaf and infused leaf. They instantly notice the variations from one Assam to the next in appearance of leaf, color of liquor and its aroma, flavour, astringency, and brightness.
http://www.gshaly.com/resources/cuppingtea.htm

"KE LAI JIN CHA" (A CUP OF TEA WILL BE BREWED)

China is known as the home town of tea.

People throughout the country drink tea daily. Because of the geographic location and climate, different places grow various kinds of tea.

In general, there are five kinds of tea classified. They are:

1. Longjin of Hangzhou,
2. Wulong of Fujian
3. Jasmine tea
4. Black tea and
5. Compressed tea.

The most conspicuous content in China's tea culture is the popular phrase when a guest arrives:

Ke Lai jin Cha meaning A cup of tea will be brewed

In the past dynasties, people not only formed a special way of tea-drinking, but also developed an **art form** called **tea-drinking**.

This art form comprises of many aspects. The most noticeable ones are:
- the making of tea
- the way of brewing
- the drinking utensils, such as a tea pot

Tea drinking is so popular in every part of the country that there is a museum especially dedicated to the tea culture in China. It is located in Hangzhou, the hometown of Longjin Tea (dragon well tea).

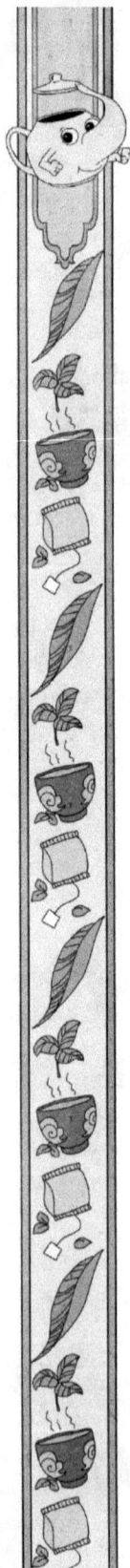

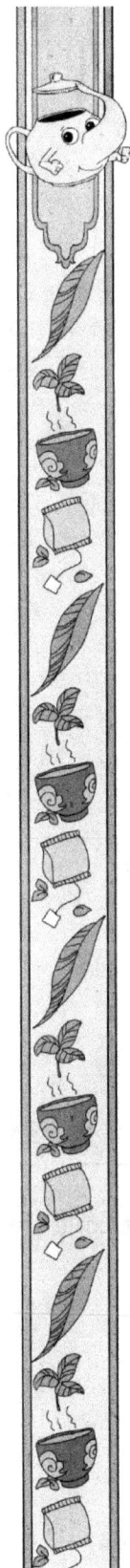

It is the only national museum of its kind. In it, there are detailed descriptions of the historic development of tea, making and brewing methods and the like.

"The China Tea Museum" is located in Shuangfeng, Longjing Road, Hangzhou, Zhejiang province.

It occupies 3.7 hectares and 8,000 square meters of construction area.

It is a national-rank museum.

The museum is clustered around tea plantations.

In side the museum, the flower corridors, fake hills, ponds and water-side pavilions are well integrated.

They have made it as a park on the southern part of the Changjiang River. Here there is a clean atmosphere and you can feel the closeness to nature.

China National Tea Museum, makes friends all over world.

http://english.teamuseum.cn

HEALING PROPERTIES OF JASMINE TEA

A cup of jasmine herbal tea is one of the most beneficial drinks that calms down your senses and helps your system to rejuvenate. It has properties that slow down the cells in the body that cause aging. It is a great drink for relieving depression, anxiety and stress.

• Jasmine Tea Balls in a Bath

In Japan, people use jasmine tea balls to take a relaxing bath after a hard day. It soothes your mind and frees your body from the day's tiredness. Even inhalation of the aroma of the jasmine tea helps the mind to calm down and releases it from stress, anxiety and tensions

Used for centuries in traditional medicine, jasmine tea has been studied in recent years for its health benefits in treating depression and other health issues. Jasmine tea is typically a blend of green tea and the jasmine flower.

The combination has a wide range of medical benefits due to the antioxidants in the tea, which help prevent heart disease and cancer. Studies also show that the use of jasmine in inhalation therapy relaxes nerves and relieves headaches.

• Aromatherapy

Never mind drinking it, just the aroma from jasmine tea has benefits.

A study published in the "European Journal of Applied Psychology" found that the inhalation of the jasmine scent produces a significant reduction in heart rate that results in a sedative effect on mood and nerve activity. Jasmine tea is widely used in aromatherapy as a stress reliever and a natural anti-depressant.

• Stroke Prevention

Medical researchers from the Chinese Academy of Medical Sciences conducted a large study with about 1000 subjects to investigate the correlation between tea consumption and stroke.

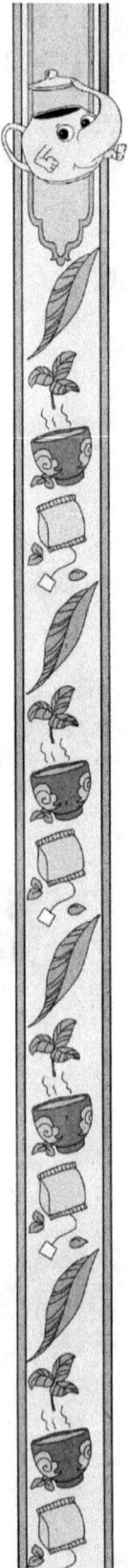

26

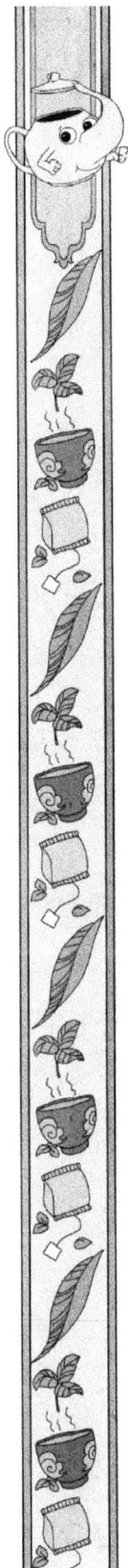

The researchers found that jasmine or green tea consumption of over 150 grams per month is statistically significant in reducing the risk of stroke. The average cup of jasmine tea contains 3.3 grams; drink two or three cups per day for stroke prevention.

• Antioxidants & Cancer

Antioxidants are molecules that protect cells against free radicals, which contributes to heart disease and cancer.

Jasmine tea is a natural polyphenol antioxidant that primarily consist of epigallocatechin gallate (EGCG). These antioxidants are absorbed in the blood when you drink jasmine tea.

Research has shown that EGCG helps treat chronic fatigue syndrome. According to the University of Maryland Center, the polyphenols found in jasmine green tea is believed to kill cancerous cells and prevent cancer.

• Lowering Cholesterol

Regularly drinking jasmine tea can help reduce cholesterol,.

To discover the effects of Chinese tea on high cholesterol, the Faculty of Medicine at the University of Hong Kong conducted a study.

Lab rats were put on a high cholesterol diet for a week and treated with different tea extracts for 8 weeks whilst maintaining the diet. The results found that green tea and jasmine tea significantly lowered serum and liver cholesterol. The high levels of the antioxidant catechin found in jasmine tea may have played a crucial role in the cholesterol reduction.

Jasmine, an herbal flowering plant, is known for its fragrance and the relaxation it promotes. Drinking herbal jasmine tea offers both health benefits and aromatherapy.

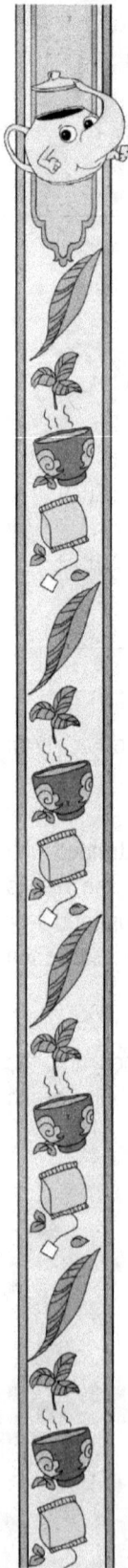

The high amounts of antioxidants found in this tea help boost your immune system and protect your body from a variety of ailments and health problem.

• Blood Sugar Regulation

Jasmine tea also helps to keep blood sugar or glucose levels balanced, according to the site www.SpiritMindBody.co.uk .

Keeping blood sugar levels can help prevent or maintain adult-onset diabetes. If you already take diabetic medications, consult your physician before drinking jasmine tea.

It may alter your blood sugar medication and cause your blood sugar to drop too low.

• Enhanced Immunity

Sipping a cup of jasmine tea, may help boost your immune system to stave off colds and infections. The antioxidant properties in this plant help your body fight off germs that normally cause you to become ill.

Drinking jasmine tea may make it more difficult for these bacteria and viruses to thrive and make you ill.

• Anti-Aging Effects

Jasmine tea may help to slow down the aging process in your body. Aging has been linked to free radicals in the body.

Jasmine tea helps to ward off these unstable molecules, protecting the walls of your cells from them. Keeping you healthy & physiologically younger.

28

CONCLUSION

I hope you have enjoyed learning or refreshing your mind about *Jasmine Tea.*

Like all tea, it certainly is beneficial to consume a certain amount of tea each day – whether it be black, green, white, herbal infusions or Oolong.

I love the many cups of tea I have each day and the variety. I have no set agenda for what I am going to have, go by what my body tells me I need at that time.

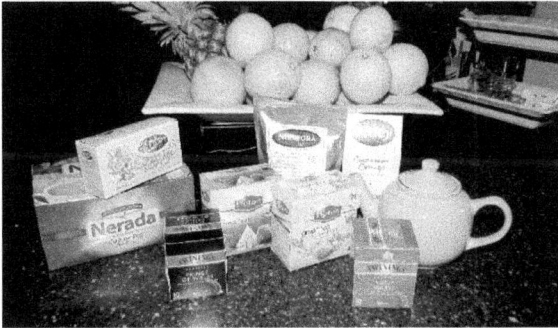

Tristan Teapot with some of the varieties of teas
we have in our panty –
plus fresh local lemons and pineapples

So enjoy your tea,
whatever it may be,

and thank you for dropping by.

ABOUT THE AUTHOR

Barbi Wildish is a writer and poet.

She loves to travel and has back-packed Australia, England, Wales, Scotland, Hong Kong, China, Vietnam, India, Thailand, Guam and Republic of Czech on her own.

When she was nineteen years old she sailed to Hong Kong and worked as a volunteer in administration and taught English to fellow workers.

She worked as a volunteer in India with a women's self-help group in administration and teaching English.

In Thailand she stayed in an Orphanage and taught the children English while completing a six weeks intensive course on 'Children At Risk'.

Also taught English in Hong Kong for two years and worked in administration in Bristol, England.

With her family Barbi has travelled to Malaysia, USA, Mexico, Italy and Israel.

She is Australian born and has travelled three-quarters of Oz's coastline fruit picking.

Barbi has had several small businesses and worked as a waitress and nurse. She currently lives with her son, his partner and their baby (2016) in Cairns, Australia.

Enjoy her easy-to-read style and be enthused to get out there, see and do and choose to be healthy and enjoy life to the full, as she does.

TRISTAN TEAPOT SERIES:

Travelling With Tristan Teapot
A TRAVEL BOOK
A journey Barbi and Tristan did in her mobile home.
They share their daily excitement & challenges
Tips about travel
A little bit of history about the towns they pass through
Healing properties of tea.

No Tea In My Cheesecake, Thank You
A RECIPE BOOK
All the recipes have *TEA* as an ingredient
Soup
Main Course
Dessert, Biscuits & Cakes
The History of Tea and
Tea Plantations in Australia

Look Out Fat, Here Comes The Green Tea
WEIGHT LOSS & CHOOSING A HEALTHIER BODY & MIND
Add Green Tea into your daily routine
All the benefits plus more
Products available to use for weight loss

To be published early 2017:

Poetry On The Way & In-Between
POEMS
From Travelling With Tristan Teapot
plus
others I have written over the years

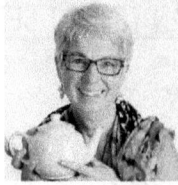

CONTACT

www.barbiwildish.com

www.facebook.com/barbiwildish

Barbi's Amazon Author's Page

Thank you for purchasing my book/s and

Don't forget:

If you have health, you have wealth

Would you kindly share my books with your friends through your social media — thank you so much

www.ingramcontent.com/pod-product-compliance
Lightning Source LLC
Chambersburg PA
CBHW060707280326
41933CB00012B/2332